Inhale Exhale

T0167710

mindful
shagging

the *calmer* sutra

POP PRESS

Inhale to the count of ten... exhale to the count of ten... in... out... in... out. Cooooooohm...

I'm Rhonda Yearn, and you might know me from TV shows such as Mindful First Dates, for my online streaming platform MindfulShags, and for founding the first mindful community of its type in the UK, a place the media described as a 'pound-shop sex cult', a criticism I observed without judgement before moving on as only the truly mindful can. In our community we practise a strict regime of mindfulness centred around the shared experience of sex. And lots of it. Seriously, come and pay us a visit some time.

Mindful shagging is the practice of bringing our awareness to this very moment in time, focusing our attention on the now as we fuck free from judgement and criticism. Sex that produces inner calm, tranquillity and self-acceptance – not to mention the best orgasms you'll ever have.

It is a discipline that requires real work and focus. No more idly looking at your phone midway through a mildly disappointing shag (unless you've both agreed to video it for MindfulShags, of course). No more wishing you'd swiped right on someone else before you ended up here. No more judging your partner for failing to hit that sexual sweet spot.

Instead you will shag like an enlightened one in the here and now, free from expectation and judgement, empowered by your thirst for inner peace and seriously satisfying sex. Your body and mind will transcend this earthly plane and take you to places you can't yet imagine, places very far from a 'pound-shop sex cult', a criticism I have definitely moved on from and am honestly fine about.

I am your guru. Your spirit guide. Your grand shag master. It's time to take you through the 60 positions handed down through centuries of mindful shagging that make up the Calmer Sutra.

Acceptance

Ommmanism

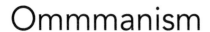

How can we discover true pleasure without first understanding how to pleasure ourselves mindfully? Focus on your breathing, channel your energy inwards, have your sex toys and tissues to hand and begin your process of self-discovery.

Because you're worth it.

Acceptance

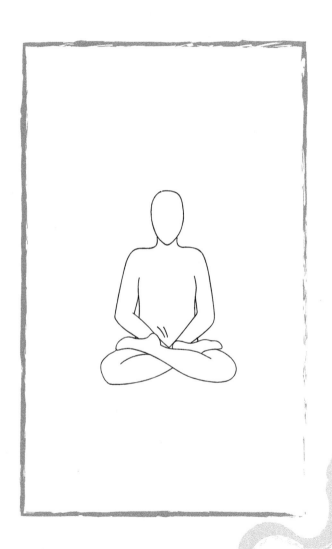

Acceptance

Lotus Lovin'

The lotus is the classic meditation pose, though what a lot of people don't realise is that its transcendental power is doubled when you throw a little hot lovin' into the mix.

Crossed legs and joined genitals make happy hearts.

Acceptance

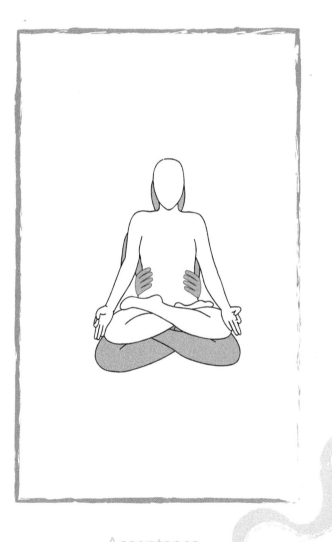

Acceptance

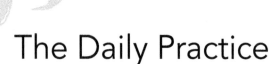

The Daily Practice

Why merely meditate when you can fornicate too? Find yourself a comfortable chair, a partner to pleasure you and make this part of your daily practice. Scientifically proven* to reduce stress and increase happiness!

*sort of

Ten minutes a day keeps the demons away.

Acceptance

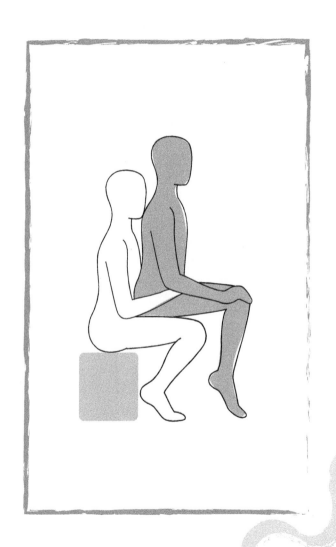

Acceptance

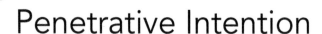

Penetrative Intention

Setting your intention is a vital part of your practice. What is your intention for this session? To be at one with the breath? To heal your mind, body and soul? Or perhaps simply to have a most excellent shag? All are valid. All are welcome.

My intention is my truth – even when I only have one intention on my mind.

Acceptance

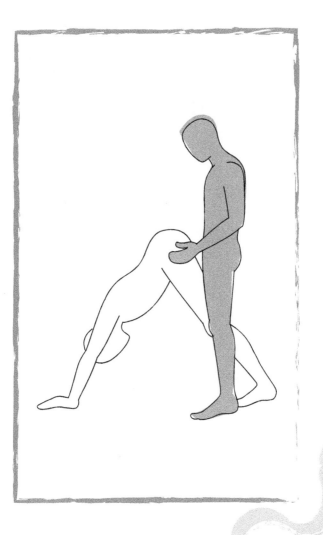

Acceptance

Wake Up

All of your life leading up to this shag has been lived on autopilot. Real life in all its technicolour glory has been going on right under your nose. It's time to Wake Up and smell the essential oils, my friend. There's no room for autopilot in this horrendously difficult position.

There are no second chances to answer the Wake Up call.

Acceptance

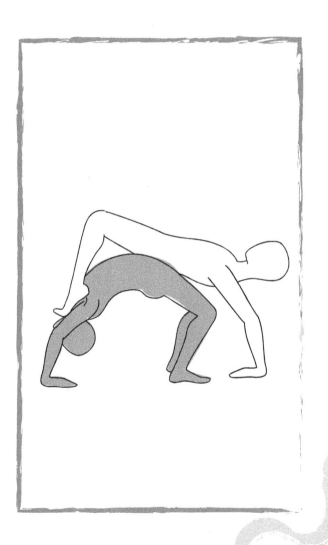

Acceptance

The Open Heart

Spread your arms wide and open up your heart to allow you to be the compassionate, empathetic human you've always been, despite some of the questionable life choices you've made in the past (no judgement here, of course). Not too wide, though – don't lose your balance!

Open heart makes loving and forgiving one's self so easy.

Acceptance

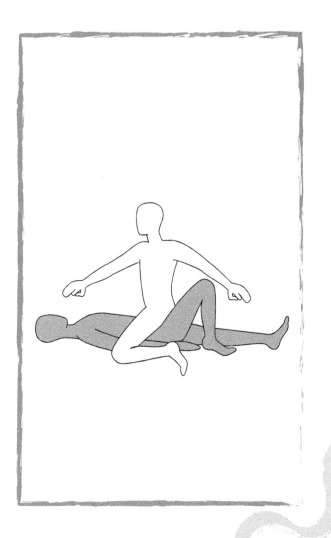

Acceptance

Let the Light In

The mind is like the weather: even on a grey and overcast day, the sun still burns brightly above the clouds. This pose opens you up to blowing away the clouds and receiving that light. Shag those unhelpful thoughts away!

I shag for the good of my body and my mind.

Acceptance

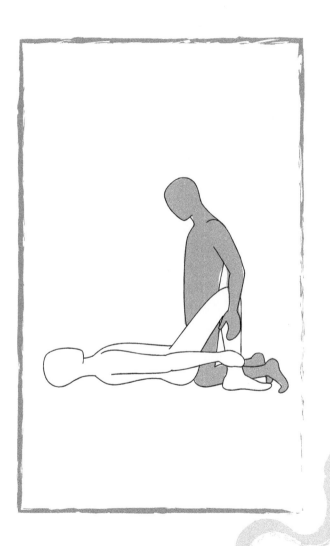

Acceptance

The Sex of Self-Acceptance

With the soles of our feet pointing skywards we can soften our gaze and look at our life clearly, free from any external pressures. Remember, everything looks better in soft focus, and everything feels better when you're shagging.

I accept myself and the lovin'
cumming my way without judgement.

Acceptance

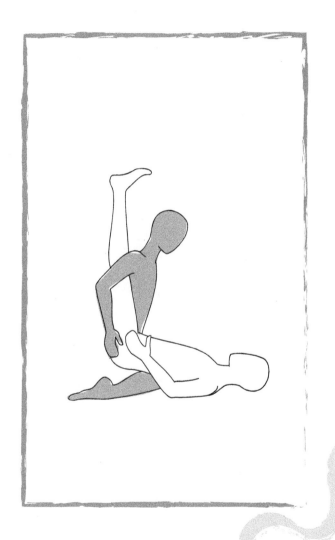

Acceptance

Grounded Grinding

Take a moment in this pose to check in with your body. Are your hands and feet grounded? Are your genitals grinding satisfactorily with the genitals of your partner? Listen to your body. Would you like to go faster, deeper, harder? Are you nearly there yet?!

Listen to your body and nourish its needs.

Acceptance

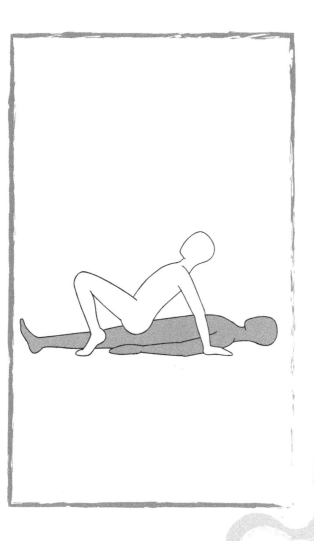

Acceptance

As the Crow Flies

Escape the shackles of this earthly plane as your crow flies high and proud. Look down at the earth. Doesn't it look small from here? See how tiny your day-to-day worries are? Congratulations – you've joined the mile-high club without even leaving the ground.

Soar through the sky then cum down to earth gently.

Acceptance

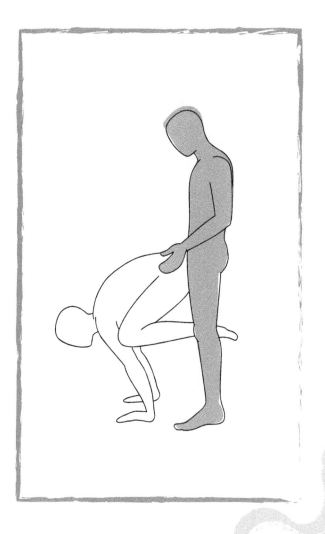

Acceptance

Crossroads

Cross your legs to symbolise the choice every Mindful Shagger must make. Down one road lies enlightenment and sexual awakening; down another lies a lifetime of TV on the sofa – watching but not seeing – and the occasional bout of joyless missionary. So what's it going to be?

Choose life. Choose Mindful Shagging.

Acceptance

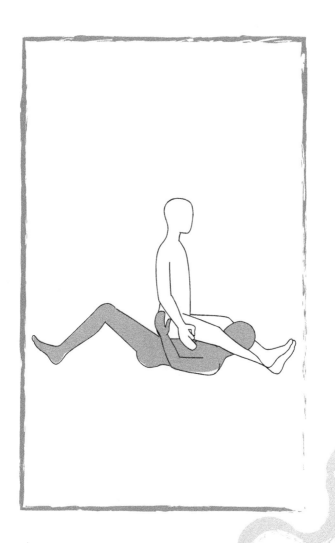

Acceptance

Trust

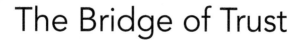

The Bridge of Trust

Meditating above an abyss offering up oral pleasure requires many years of practice to make perfect. Make sure your roots are strong so that, at the moment of climax, you judder as if in an earthquake, but your bridge does not collapse.

I'm structurally sound so let oral pleasure abound.

Trust

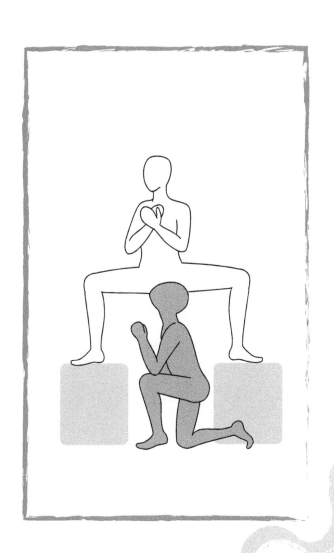

Trust

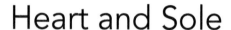

Heart and Sole

Feet meet heart, heart meet feet. Connect these rarely aligned body parts and discover what it's like to be the ground beneath your partner's feet. With heart and sole aligned the promise of deep penetration and spiritual connection is assured.

Feet to heart centre, I'm ready to enter.

Trust

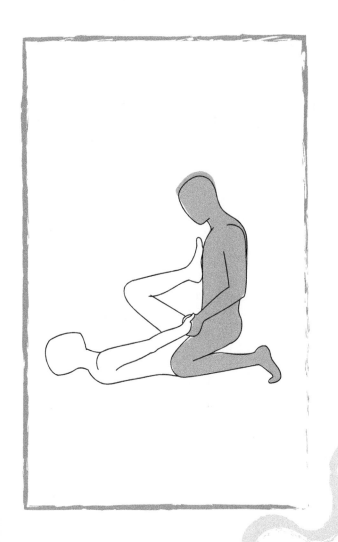

Trust

Inverting the Shag

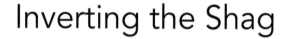

Send your blood flowing to the hungriest organ of them all – the mind, of course – while your partner takes care of another organ in need of some serious nourishment. Take a moment to check in with your body and appreciate what having the world turned upside down is like.

It takes an inversion to tame my perversion.

Trust

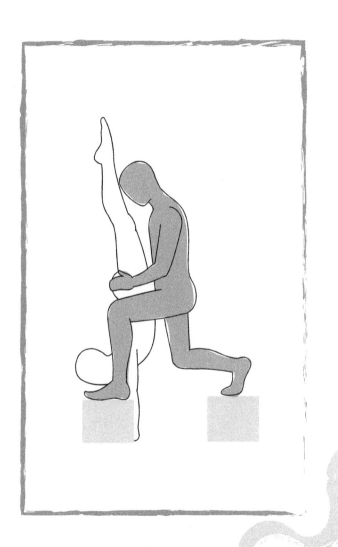

Trust

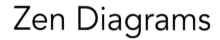

Zen Diagrams

'When you drink just drink; when you shag just shag' goes the ancient Zen saying – or something like that, anyway – but given that a picture paints a thousand words, why not find the point of intersection with your partner and shag your way through an easy-to-follow Zen Diagram.

When you shag, just shag (following this diagram).

Trust

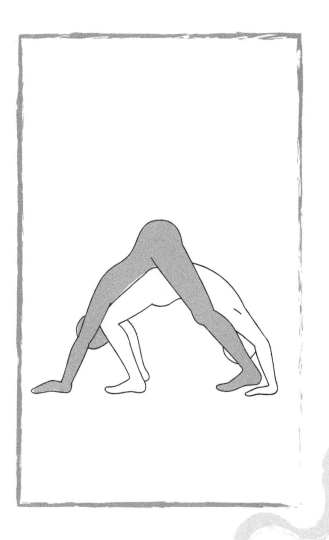

Trust

Mindful Mirror

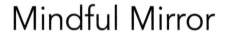

Mindful shagging isn't just about the destination – it's about the journey too. Mirror your partner's pose, join your bodies together and share your sexual energy as you travel along your road of enlightenment, making sure to arrive at your destination at the same time.

Mirror, mirror on the wall, observe me without judgement, that's all.

Trust

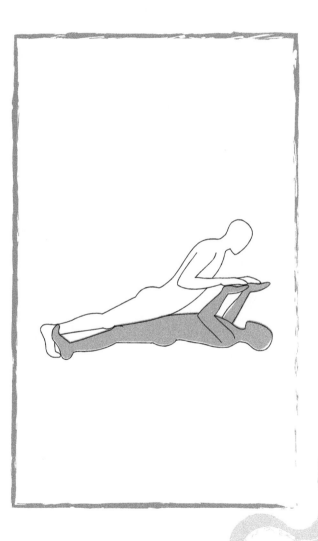

Trust

The Squat of Delight

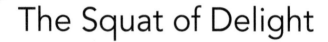

'She (or he) who doth squat, doth controleth the rhythm of the world' sayeth the ancient Mindful Shagging scrolls. Which basically means the person squatting is in charge, so just sit still and enjoy the delightful ride.

Before the might of your squat,
I'll cum quite a lot.

Trust

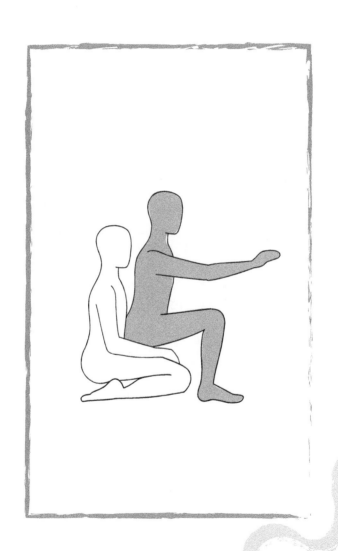

Trust

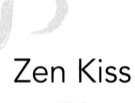

Zen Kiss

Pucker up for a Zen Kiss and understand just how interconnected our energies are. Observe the feelings in your lips, your tongue – the tingling, moist sensations. Be playful. Be present. And yeah, you might as well shag while you're there.

Our lips are the energy centres of our intertwined beings.

Trust

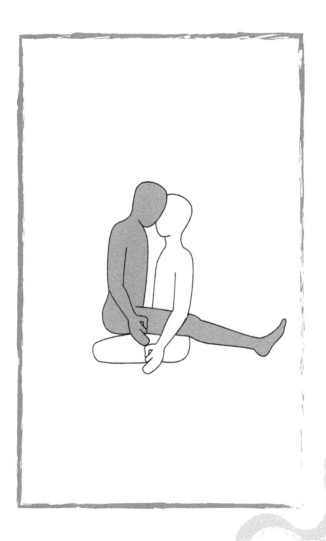

Trust

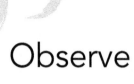

Observe

Observe your partner's back as if for the first time. Look at the rise and fall of their breath; examine each individual vertebrae along their spine; read the undulations of their skin like a map. Wait, you are still aroused, right? Get shagging!

Your body's a map I long to get lost in.

Trust

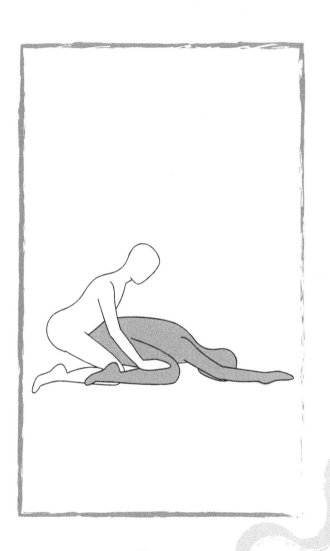

Trust

The Cradle of Calm

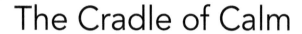

The Cradle of Calm is every Mindful Shagger's refuge from the frenzy of the modern world, a sanctuary of slow, dreamy sex and maybe just a smidgen of lower-back and hamstring ache to be acknowledged without judgement.

Keep to the Cradle and the real world seems like a fable

Trust

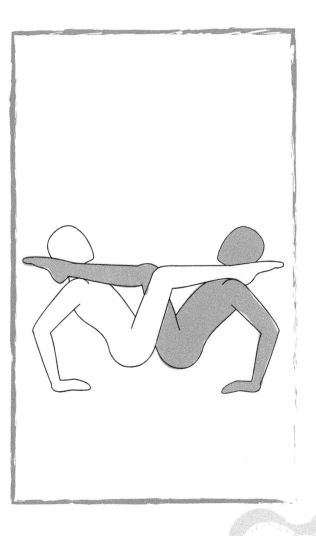

Trust

Lovers' Lock

Securing your lover in the Lovers' Lock and throwing away the metaphorical key allows you to mindfully explore one another, free from any distractions of the outside world. Only once you are fully satisfied should you release your lover. (Safe word to be agreed beforehand.)

I have you under lock and key;
I'll decide when you go free.

Trust

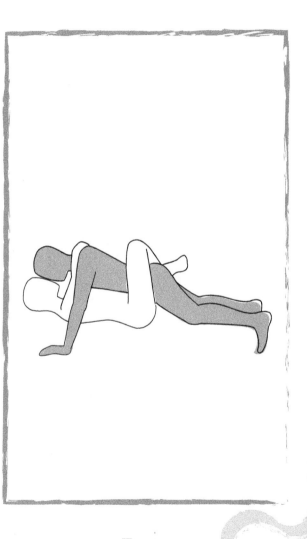

Trust

Mindful Hair

Penetrating your partner from behind, run your hands through their hair, being truly present and absorbing the texture, the way it falls, its colour in the light. If they're bald, that's fine. Just give their head a mindful rub.

Hair, scalp, body, mind – all as one, all real fine.

Trust

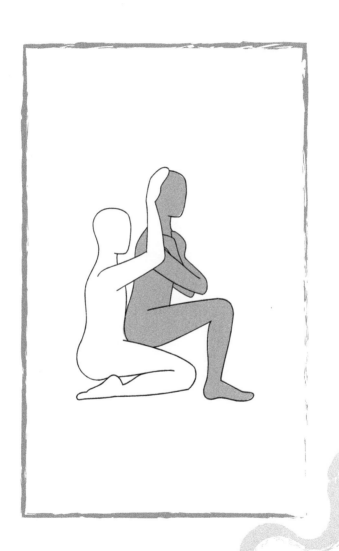

Trust

Generosity

Mindful Rimming

Synchronising one's breath to match the rhythm of both hand- and rim-job takes some doing, but that's why we talk about your 'practice' when it comes to Mindful Shagging. So what are you waiting for? Get practising!

My cup floweth over when its rim is awoken.

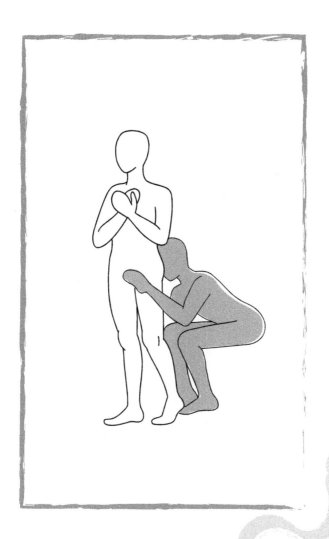

Generosity

The Breath of Pleasure

Oral pleasure can only be truly given wholly once one has learned to accept one's self and make sexual offerings free of ego. Having said that, in order to achieve spiritual harmony it is only fair that one's partner returns the favour tout de suite.

I breathe for your pleasure; soon you will breathe for mine.

Generosity

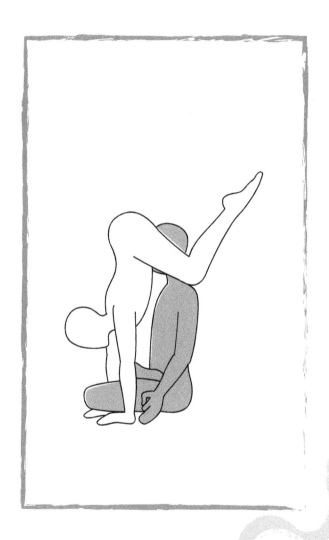

Generosity

The Deeper Question

Your partner is exposed before you. Lower yourself slowly, inch by inch upon them. Inhale. Exhale. Find that sweet, sweet spot and ride yourself to the kind of climax that gives space to the deeper questions in life, such as, 'When can we do that again?'

Self-control is king on the expedition to answer the Deeper Question.

Generosity

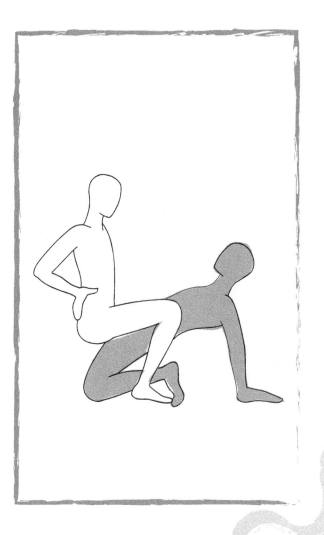

Generosity

The Present's Present

Yesterday is gone. Tomorrow never knows. The present is the only gift we can truly enjoy. So observe without judgement. Bring your awareness back to the breath. Be kind. Be curious. Be sexy. Now get shagging in the moment – that's the present's greatest gift of all.

How do you like me now
(and only now)?!

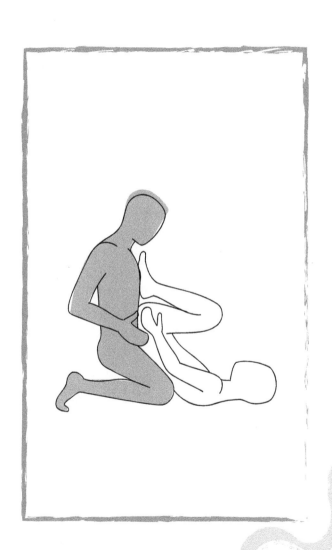

Generosity

The Sensual Serpent

Indulge in some serious self-care by burning sage and then deliver pleasure with your darting, serpentine tongue, while entwined with your partner and maintaining control of your breath. If you don't have any sage, don't worry about it.

Sage is the healer and the sexy herb.

Generosity

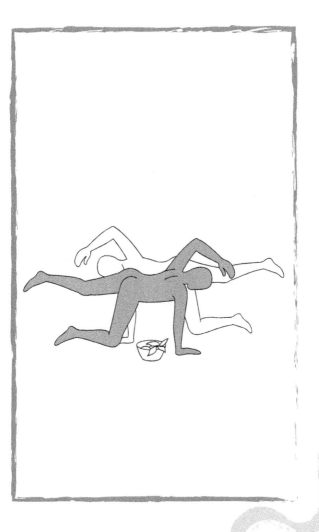

Generosity

Zen 69

Search for the true meaning of life through the giving and receiving of oral pleasure. Absorb your partner's energy while they absorb yours in a virtuous circle. Make it part of your practice to aspire to the divine light – the simultaneous orgasm, pure giving-and-receiving nirvana.

The desire for self-knowledge stirs first in the loins.

Generosity

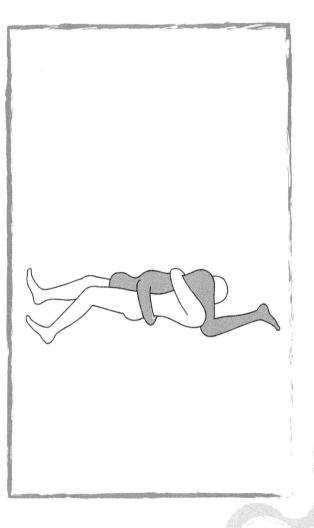

Generosity

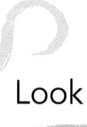

Look

You look – hell, yeah – but do you see? Lock eyes with your partner, block out all other senses and drive each other wild merely through looking at each other. OK, fine, you can masturbate – just do it mindfully.

Beauty is in the third eye of the beholder.

Generosity

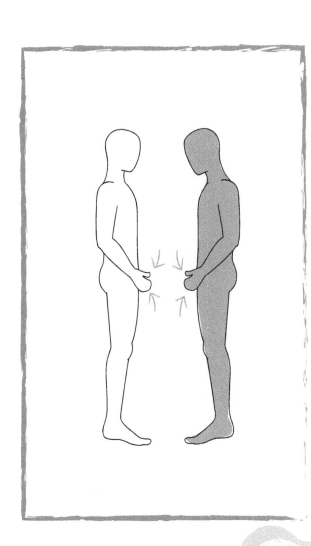

Generosity

Taste

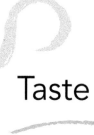

I want you to really explore the sensation of taste. No, don't just say 'it's a bit metallic'. Don't tell me what your last meal was. FFS, I don't mean 'spit or swallow'! Let's really explore this sense in granular detail while you deliver mindful pleasure to your partner.

Taste buds are my teammates in mindful pleasure.

Generosity

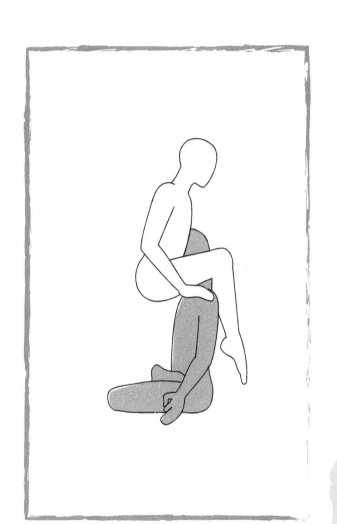

Generosity

Feel

Close your eyes and shut down all senses except the sense of touch. How does their body feel pressed up against yours? Move your hands all over their body and observe how that really feels, free from judgement. If you feel your mind wander, return to your breath – and your thrusts.

Close your eyes and just feel – you know it's unreal!

Generosity

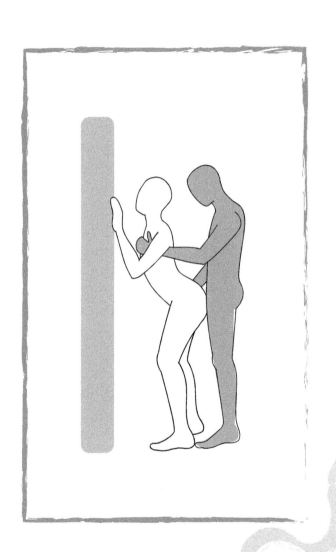

Generosity

Breeze Dangle

Bend forward and let it all go. Take a moment to connect with that sensation of freedom, offering no resistance as your body undulates to the rhythm of the pleasure from your partner. You are a small, connected part of the vast universe, you beautiful mindful thing you.

I'm a willow dangling in the breeze, free to do all that I please.

Generosity

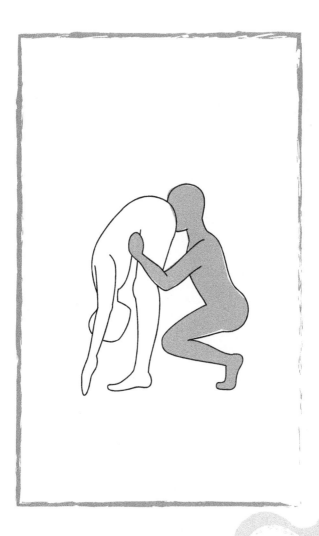

Generosity

Mindful Fingers

Bring your attention to your hands and fingers. Explore every little sensation down to the tips of your fingers, while your partner explores every little sensation your hands are creating on their body. It's a reach-around, sure, but mindfully done.

Mindful fingers make light of hard work.

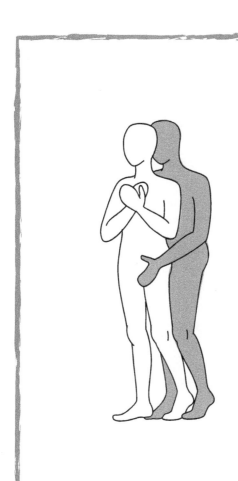

Generosity

Patience

Passing Clouds

Inhale, exhale. In, out. Align your strokes
with your breath so that you function as one
smooth-operating machine. Inhale slowly,
exhale slowly… it takes supreme command
of your being not to lose control of your
breath and pant your way speedily to
the climax!

Passing clouds are in no rush,
so why am I?

Patience

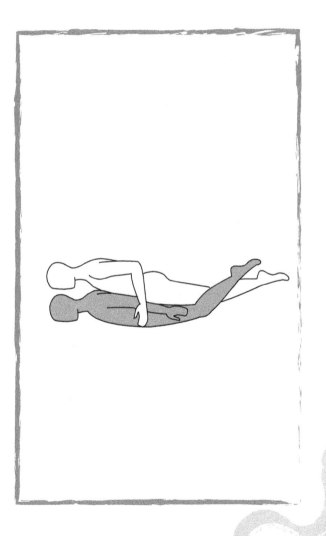

Patience

Perfect Practice

A practice you can turn to anywhere, whether it's a park, at home or in a public toilet. Observe your surroundings mindfully. Really hear the song of that bird. Seriously smell the perfume of that flower. Truly see the colour of that graffiti promising 'fun times' by dialling its number.

Practice can be made perfect wherever there's a warm and willing body beside you.

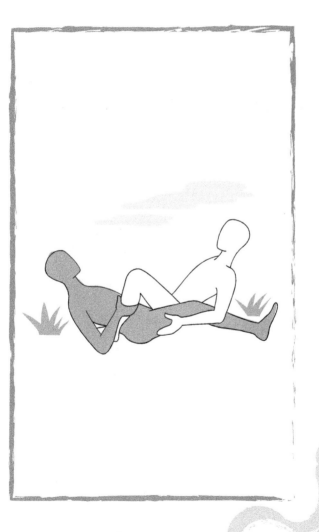

Patience

Labour of Lovin'

A position that requires physical exertion but which allows your mind, in contrast, to remain calm and at peace. Observe your efforts to hold your partner and shag them. Send the breath to where your body cries out for it. And for mindful fuck's sake, don't drop your partner!

My body's toils won't make my mind recoil.

Patience

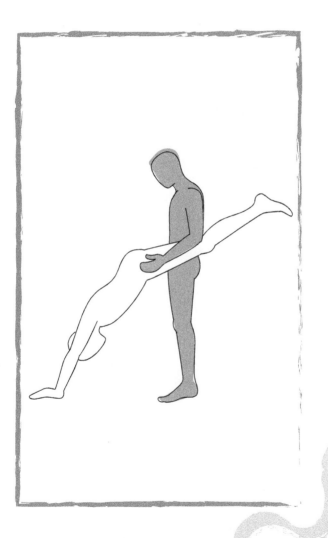

Patience

The Letting Go

Shag mindfully and then, with the finishing line in sight, let go of it all. Let your breath run wild, your mind drift to wherever it may choose and just let. It. All. Go. Liberating, isn't it? But don't indulge it too long – get back to observing every damn sound and sight and smell again quick-smart.

To be truly mindful one must first learn when not to be mindful.

Patience

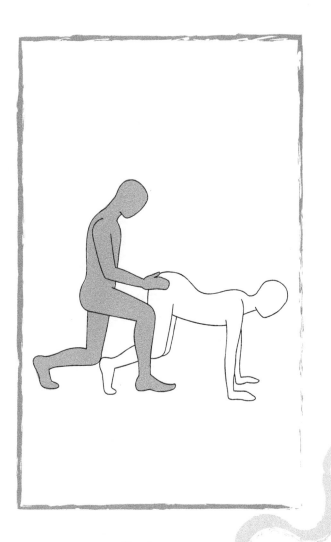

Patience

The Body Scan

Scan your body from head to toe, checking in with each part of your body. How does your head feel? Your chest? Your tummy? Many new practitioners fail to get past their genitals and find themselves racing to the promised land, but with practice comes control. You'll get down to your toes one day.

I'll scan my body if you scan yours?

Patience

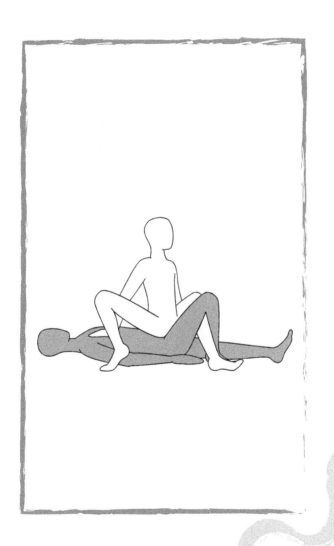

Patience

Sensual Slow Down

In today's frantic and frenetic world, it can be difficult to find a moment's peace. Turn back the clocks. Dial it down to half speed. Let's do it low and slow. Turn that two-minute shag into a two-hour marathon and watch your worries drift away like passing clouds.

No need for worry so long as you're not in a hurry.

Patience

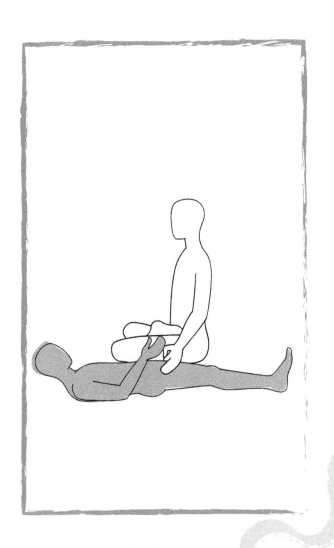

Patience

The Rise and Fall

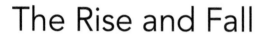

Bring your attention to the rise and fall of your chest and belly, while you admire the chest and belly of your partner – if that's your sort of thing, of course. Maybe you're more a legs and bum type? And then slowly bring your attention to the rise and fall of your hips and shag them senseless, mindfully speaking of course.

Seek your pleasure at your own leisure.

Patience

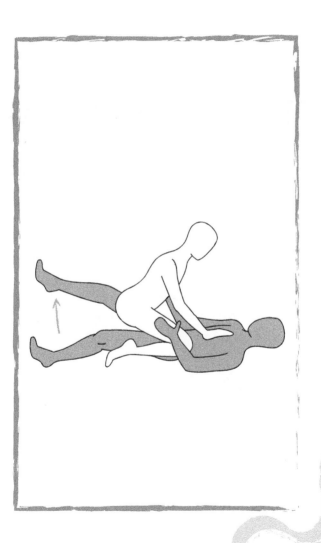

Patience

The Pleasure in Stillness

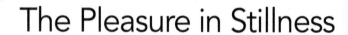

Shoulders should be relaxed and mind clear if we are to hold this pose. Observe the present moment. How do you feel at this precise point in time? Don't get distracted by what you are doing later or what you had for breakfast – even if this is your go-to technique for avoiding premature ejaculation. There is no judgement in Mindful Shagging.

Life's pressures may come and go, but I will continue to cum and blow.

Patience

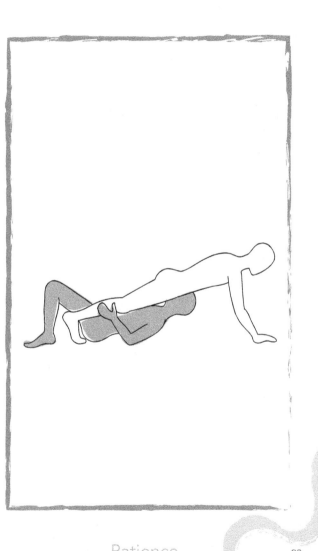

Patience

Pigeon Power

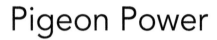

This powerful yogic hip opener also helps open up other areas down there too, which allows for intense penetration that is almost certainly not for beginners. Open your mind to the power of the winged scavenger.

Fly like a pigeon, cum like a river.

Patience

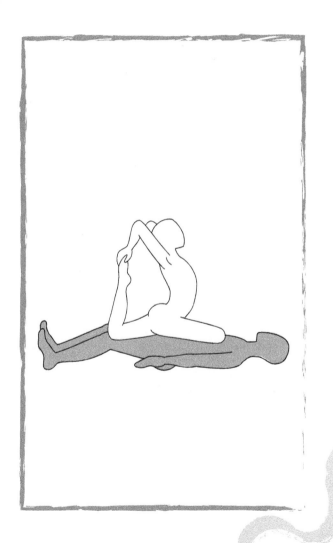

Patience

Patient Pleasures

A pose that rewards patience and no little effort in order to achieve perfect alignment with your partner, the pleasure you'll derive as you fuck freely in the here and now will provide its own enlightenment.

I'm in no hurry to reach my road's end: the journey itself is my destination.

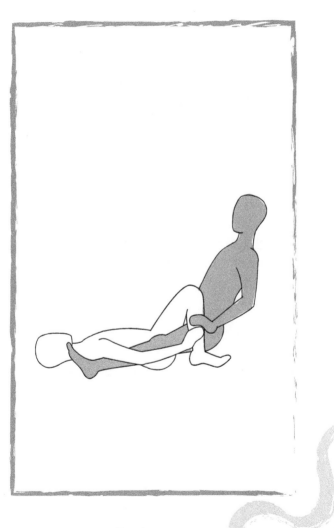

Patience

Tree in Wind

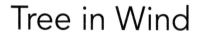

Filter out all sounds except for the wind whistling through the nearby willows. That's nature. That's the present. Now, I want you to be that tree, bending elegantly in the wind. No, the tree isn't getting shagged. That's just you.

Whenever the wind blows me,
I'm happy.

Patience

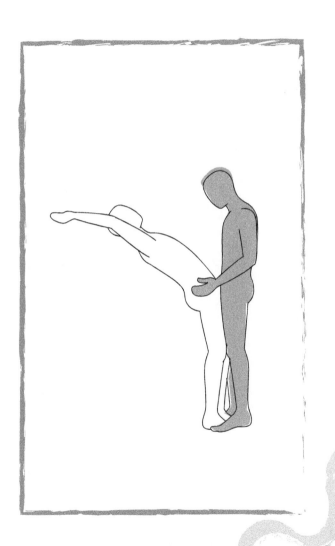

Patience

Scent

A much-underrated sense in the bedroom, but as long as you both have a tolerable hygiene regime, shutting out the other senses and getting intoxicated on the scent of your lover is a mindful experience that can convert even the most sceptical guest of your sex cult.

Inhale deeply… you smell gorgeous, my pretty.

Patience

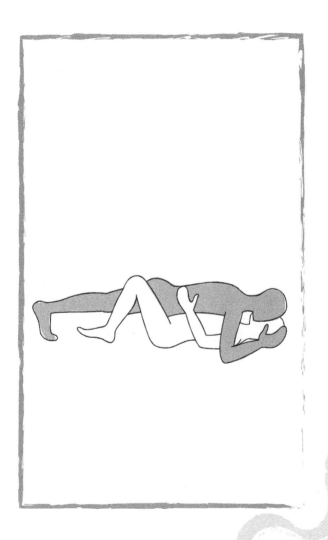

Patience

Gratitude

Meditation Levitation

Meditation can make you levitate – though you will almost certainly need a sexual organ inside you to do so. Meditate your way through the sky while maintaining an attitude of gratitude towards your partner for allowing you to soar so high.

Meditate, penetrate, levitate!

Gratitude

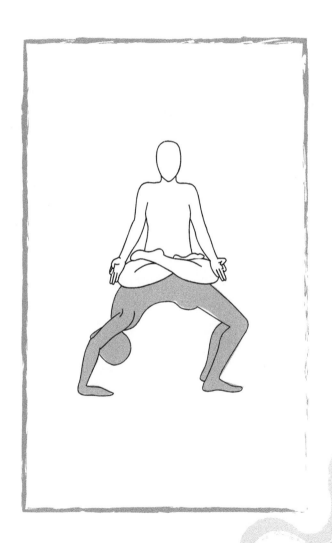

Gratitude

Finishing-off Pose

Lie back and allow your body and mind to completely relax. Slow the breath down and check in with your body patiently and with gratitude. Thank yourself for your practice. Thank your partner for the blow job.

What is done is done. What must cum will cum.

Gratitude

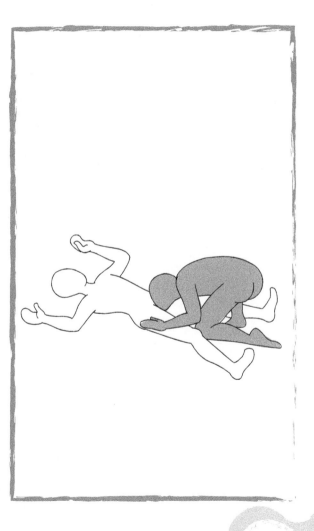

Gratitude

The Wheel of Gratitude

Maintaining the wheel can be difficult on the body, but it is important to ride this line between pleasure and pain, to accept without judgement that we might struggle in this position and yet give thanks that we too are receiving oral pleasure.

Thank you, thank you, thank you!

Gratitude

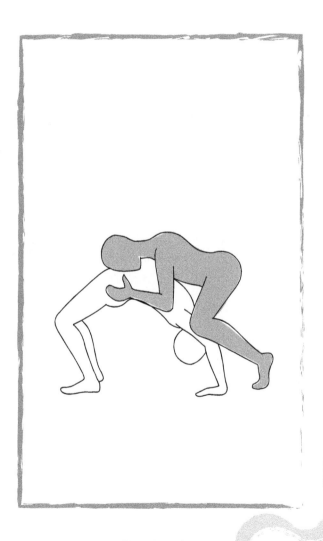

Gratitude

Prayer Pose

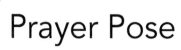

Pray while your partner kneels before you. Keep your body straight and still. Feel your breath. Feel their breath. There is nothing outside of this present moment in time. This might just be a spiritual experience.

I pray to the mindful gods and I pray to the gods of sexual healing

Gratitude

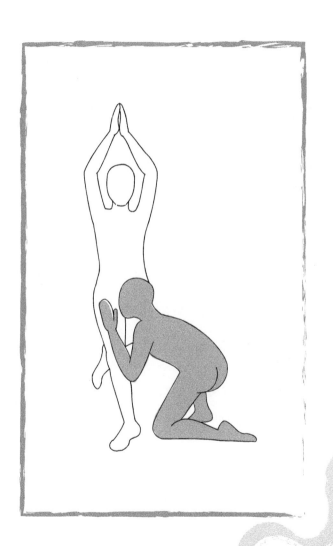

Gratitude

The Air of Enlightenment

Allow your feet to lift off the ground and give thanks to your partner for offering themselves so fully for your pleasure. Only this high can the air feel so rarefied and full of possibility. Of course, the best way to give thanks to your partner is to give them a shag they'll never forget.

The road to enlightenment is paved with hot, sweating, naked flesh.

Gratitude

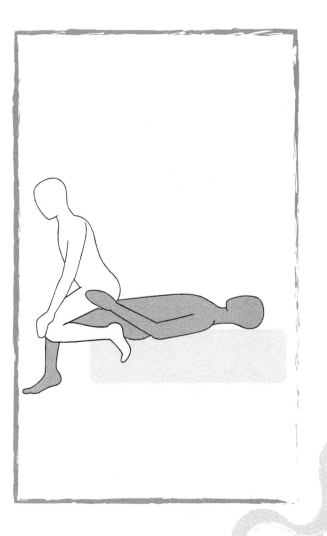

Gratitude

The Big O

That's Ommm, of course, though you're hardly going to be judged for indulging in a screaming, body-trembling orgasm while you chant. That's just not the mindful way. But be sure to resume chanting your Ommms as soon as possible. Even if it's just to say, 'Ommm, that's me done, thanks.'

Ommmmmmmmmmmmmmmmm…

Gratitude

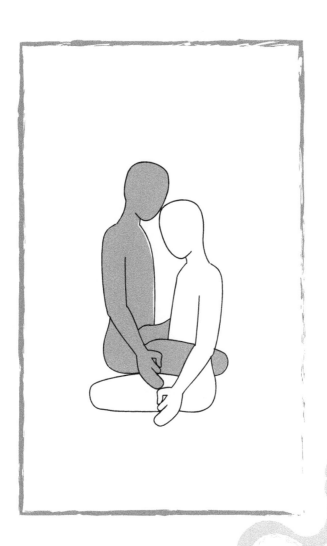

Gratitude

Giving-head Space

Your Giving-head Space gives you the opportunity to check in with all aspects of your body. How do your legs and arms feel? Your chest, your back? And that mouth on your genitals – how does *that* feel?

Open legs are the key to an open mind.

Gratitude

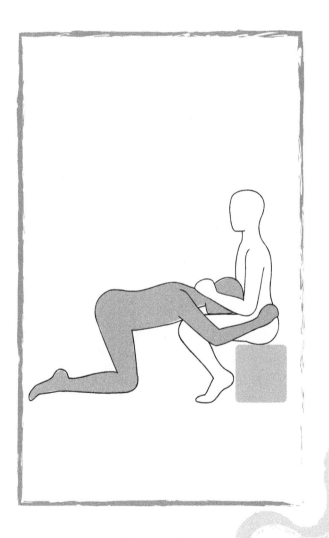

Gratitude

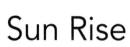

Sun Rise

The sun isn't the only thing sure to rise as you shag eastwards. Your feelings of calm and alignment with the earth's planetary rhythms will simply soar, darling!
Good morning!

Look to the east and soothe the inner beast.

Gratitude

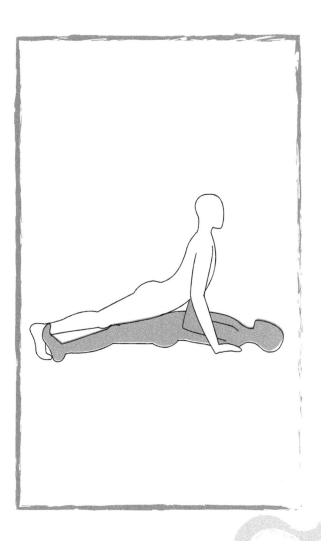

Gratitude

Sun Set

A sun-downer session provides ample opportunity to express your gratitude for the day that's just been. The sun in the sky. The food on your table. The hot body panting towards climax beneath you. Here's to fucking gratitude.

West is best for some end-of-day lovin'.

Gratitude

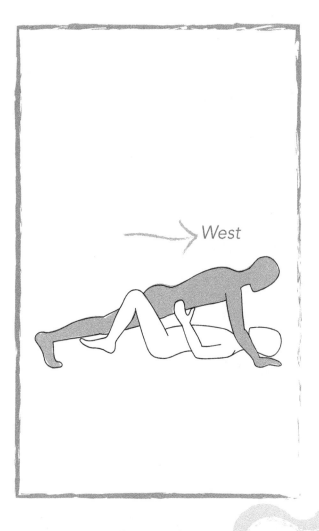

West

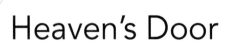

Heaven's Door

Reach for the sky as your partner feels for your depths. Inhale… exhale… And when the inevitable happens, just go with it and allow the heavens to finally open.

Worldly pleasures won't pass me by as I touch the sky.

Gratitude

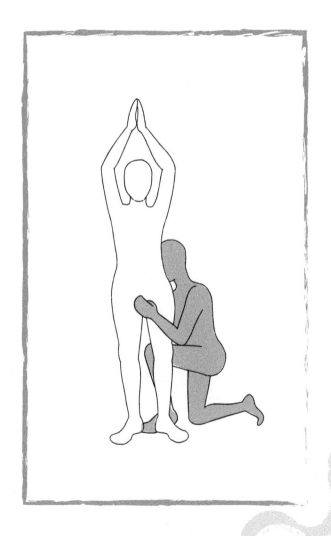

Gratitude

Inner Peace/
Outer Chaos

Cast off your inhibitions and go wild with lust – but inside remain mindful. Be grateful. Be of one with the breath. Be open to all senses. Be ready to… cooohm!

Only in the eye of chaos can we hope to find calm.

Gratitude

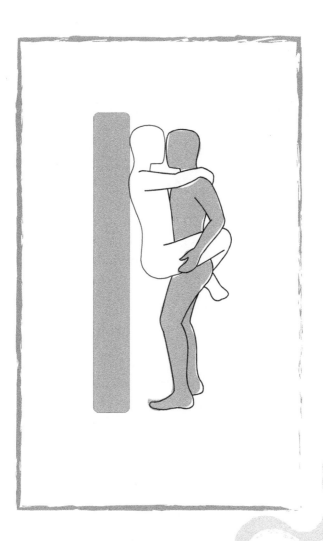

Gratitude

Listen

You listen but do you truly hear? Pour all your attention into this one sense, listening to the beat of your partner's heart, the rise and fall of their breath while you give them a hand job. Speed up, slow down. Tease. But make sure you really hear, not merely listen.

Those who listen sometimes cannot hear without the power of Mindful Shagging.

Gratitude

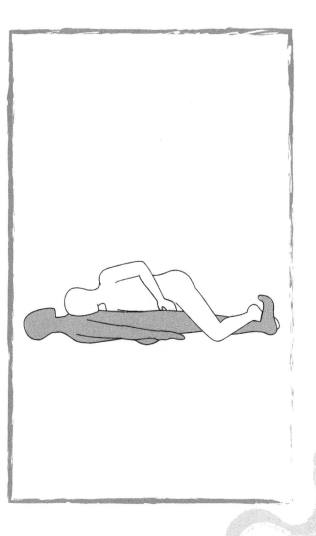

Gratitude

2

Pop Press, an imprint of Ebury Publishing,
20 Vauxhall Bridge Road,
London SW1V 2SA

Pop Press is part of the Penguin Random House group of companies
whose addresses can be found at global.penguinrandomhouse.com

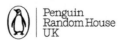

Penguin
Random House
UK

Copyright © Pop Press 2020

First published in the United Kingdom by Pop Press in 2020

www.penguin.co.uk

A CIP catalogue record for this book is available from the
British Library

ISBN 9781529107166

Design by Emily Snape
Copywriter: Steve Burdett
Project management by whitefox

Printed and bound in Great Britain by Clays Ltd, Elcograf S.p.A.

Penguin Random House is committed to a sustainable future for our
business, our readers and our planet. This book is made from Forest
Stewardship Council® certified paper.

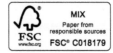